Evolution of Bambusa Arundinacea

Includes Cases and Practical Understanding

Emily Goodman,
Classical Homeopath

Dedication

This book is dedicated to my loving husband, whose unlimited support and encouragement made this book possible. Thank you so much for constantly encouraging me.

Also a special thanks to my father-in-law, mother-in-law and my parents for their endless support and encouragement.

TABLE OF CONTENTS

Chapter 1: Introduction to Bamboo Tree

Introduction

This chapter is focused on the introduction of Bamboo tree. This chapter describes the properties, and the uses of Bamboo tree in various culture and in various part of the world.

The properties of Bamboo tree will help to understand the key features and core of Bambusa, a homeopathic remedy derived from Bamboo tree especially temperate woody Bamboos (type of Bamboo species – Bamboo Arundinacea). Even though most of us are aware about the importance of this tree, we will explore the deeper aspects of Bamboo tree

Let's understand some features of Bamboo tree.

Properties and Features of Bamboo Tree

Flexibility and Elasticity: Bamboo tree has an ability to grow quickly than any other tree. Based on the size and girth you would never guess that this tree is one of the strongest tree. But what's amazing about the bamboo tree is its flexibility and elasticity nature. When the wind reaches 100 mph and there's tropical storms, hurricanes, and typhoons the bamboo tree will bend all the way down to the ground! Sometimes less than inch off the ground but someway will bounce back!! So much is the flexibility and elasticity of this tree. Hence Bamboo tree is best known for its ability to bend but not break.

Continuous growth: Bamboo trees have amazing potential for growth, however its growth is not noticeable.

Strong: The body of a single bamboo tree is not large by any means when compared to the other much larger trees in the forest. It may not look impressive at first sight at all. But the plants endure cold winters and extremely hot summers and are sometimes the only trees left standing in the aftermath of a typhoon. They may not reach the heights of the other trees, but they are strong and stand tall in extreme weather. Bamboo is not as fragile as it may appear, not by a long shot.

Distribution and Ecology of Bamboo Tree

Bamboos are the fastest-growing plants in the world, with growth rate of 250cm in 24 hours noted. However the growth rate depends on the condition of soil and climate as it grows rapidly in temperate climatic conditions.

Certain species of bamboo can grow 91 cm (3 ft) within a 24-hour period, at a rate of almost 4 cm (1.5 in) an hour (a growth around 1 mm every 40 seconds, or one inch every 40 minutes). Unlike all other trees, the stem of individual Bamboo tree emerge from the ground and grow to their full height in a single growing season of 3 to 4 months. During these months, each new shoot grows vertically into a culm (stem) with no branching out until the majority of the mature height is reached. Then, the branches extends and leafing out occurs.

Bamboos are of notable economic and cultural significance in South Asia, Southeast Asia and East Asia, being used for building materials, as a food source, and as a versatile raw product. Bamboo has a higher compressive strength than wood, brick, or concrete and a tensile strength that rivals steel.

Bamboo species are found in the diverse climate, especially in East Asia, Northern Australia, West India, Sub-Saharan Africa and Mid-Atlantic States of America.

The temperate Bamboo species can survive temperature as low as -29 degree C while other bamboo species die at or near freezing temperatures.

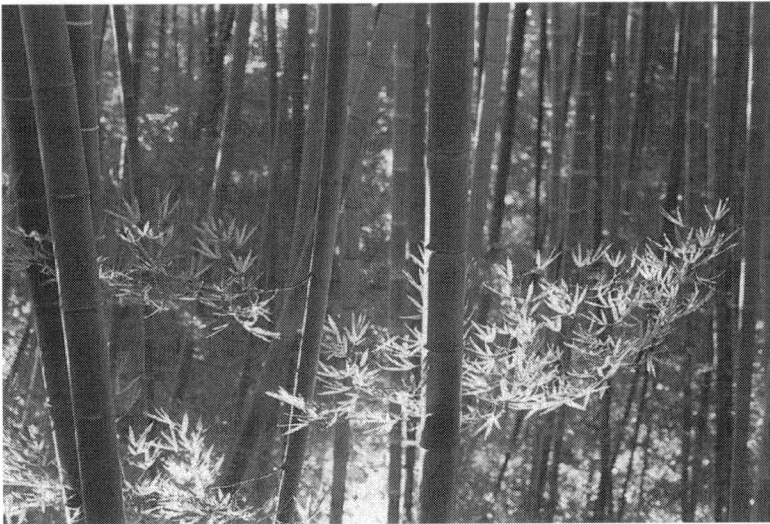

Bamboo Tree

Uses of Bamboo in some culture

- Culinary use:
  a. The shoots of Bamboo is used in numerous Asian dishes and broths, and are available in supermarkets in various sliced forms, in both fresh and canned versions.
  b. Bamboo leaves are used as wrappers for steamed dumplings with rice and other ingredients.
  c. Many Nepalis and Indians prepare delicacies from fresh Bamboo shoots.
  d. In many culture, Bamboo are used for cooking utensils and is also used in manufacture of chopsticks.

- Medicinal use:

  a. In Chinese medicine, Bamboo are used for treating infections and general healing of body.

  b. Tabasheer is one of the main substances from bamboo used in Ayurvedic and Tibetan medicine and it is called as bamboo-manna or bamboo silica (because it is rich in silica). This substance has certain properties like stimulant, astringent, febrifuge, tonic, antispasmodic, and aphrodisiac. An Ayurvedic remedy, Sitopaladi Churna which is a powder made with tahasheer as amain ingredient was used traditionally for tuberculosis and other wasting diseases and has been adopted as a popular remedy for common cold, sore throat, sinus congestion, and cough. In Tibet, formulas with Tabasheer as the main ingredient are used for treating lung diseases.

- Construction use:

    a. In Asia and South America, Bamboos are traditionally been used as the construction material.

    b. Bamboo was used for structural members of the India Pavilion at Expo 2010 in Shanghai. Pavilion is the largest bamboo dome, with the total of 30 km (19 mi) of bamboo was used. The dome is supported on 18-m-long steel piles and a series of steel ring beams. The bamboo was treated with borax and boric acid as a fire retardant and insecticide and bent in the required shape. The bamboo sections were joined with reinforcement bars and concrete mortar to achieve the necessary lengths.

- Other uses:

    a. Bamboo pulps are mainly produced in China, Myanmar, Thailand, and India, and are used in printing and writing papers.

    b. Bamboo is used for crafting the bows and arrows used in the Japanese martial art.

    c. Many musical instruments like flute are made from Bamboo wood.

Conclusion

'Bend but does not break' describes the nature of Bamboo tree.

Bamboo tree has been used since many years in different cultures.

References:

Wikipedia. https://en.wikipedia.org/wiki/Bamboo.

Chapter 2: Core of Bambusa Arundinacea

In this chapter we will learn the theme or core of Bambusa Arundinacea. Understanding of the core of remedy will help to differentiate the remedy from the other similar ones and also help to understand the whole picture of the remedy.

CANNOT STAND ALONE and WANT OF SUPPORT is the core of Bambusa remedy. 'Bend but does not break' is a type of personality.

If you visualize the appearance of Bamboo, they grow in clusters, you will never see Bamboo plant growing in single. They cannot grow alone as they need support and company all the time. There is need of physical and mental support to function well.

Bamboo tree contains a substance called ' Tabasheer' present at the nodal joints of Bamboo. This substance is composed of water and silica, with traces of lime, and potash. Hence this plant is closely aligned with the mineral silica for want of support.

The main action of this remedy is on the back, neck, shoulders, and extremities. Also it is useful during child birth and pregnancy. Stiffness of the muscles is the main and most important symptom.

Important Rubrics of Bambusa

Let's go in depth and understand the core of this remedy. Following are the general and mental rubrics of Bambusa Arundinacea taken from Synthesis repertory.

- Anxiety conscience
- Ailments from honor wounded
- Ailments from emotional
- Ailments from anger suppressed
- Ailments from anticipation
- Carried desire to be
- Change desire to be
- Cheerful
- Concentration difficult
- Confidence want of confidence, failure feels himself to be
- Confidence want of self-confidence, support desires
- Discontented himself
- Delusion alone being in the world
- Delusions arms stiff
- Delusion life cut off
- Delusion back loosened, back is
- Delusion back packed in streaks of fog; back is
- Delusion fail everything will
- Delusion forsaken
- Delusion, health he has ruined with
- Delusion meaningless everything he is
- Delusion poor he is
- Delusion soul something presses on her
- Delusion, succeed, everything he does wrong, he cannot.
- Delusion, symptoms comes outside of his

- Delusion, tired
- Delusion soul something presses her
- Delusion wrong, everything goes wrong
- Despair death, fear of, with
- Despair death fear of with – separate him with children, death will
- Despair, destiny everything is controlled by
- Despair supported wants to be
- Disturbed aversion to be
- Dullness
- Ennui, laziness with
- Fear – disease, cancer, convulsion, disease impending of
- Fear of Failure
- Fear of narrow spaces
- Helpless feeling of
- Irritability
- Indifference everything to
- Indifference joy of other
- Indifference mental exertion during
- Laziness sadness from
- Loquacity
- Loathing
- Light desire for
- Offended easily
- Postponing
- Prostration of mind
- Quiet wants to be
- Responsibility aversion to
- Responsibility taking too seriously
- Sadness, occupation amel
- Sadness menses before
- Sadness aversion to company, desire solitude

- Sensitive reprimands to
- Slowness
- Tension mental
- Weeping, forsaken feeling from
- Weeping while telling sickness to
- Confidence, want of self-confidence, failure feels himself a
- Confidence, want of self-confidence, plans about realizing her
- Confidence, want of self-confidence, support desire
- Yielding disposition
- Back stiffness, painful
- Back stiffness, cold agg
- Back stiffness, rising, stopping from
- Back Stiffness, motion amel
- Back Stiffness, cervical region, turning head agg
- Back Stiffness warmth amel
- Back, stiffness, cervical region, weather, change of weather
- Extremities, coldness.
- Extremities, formication
- Extremities, Numbness
- Extremities, pain, wandering, stitching pain
- Extremities, pain, waves in
- Extremities pain, appear suddenly disappear suddenly
- Sleep, interrupted
- Sleep, restless
- Sleep, sleeplessness, midnight at
- Sleep, sleeplessness- mental tension from
- Sleep, sleeplessness, thoughts, activity of thoughts from
- Sleep, waking frequently

- Dreams, water of
- Generals, open air, desire for open air
- Generals, cold agg

Above mentioned rubrics will help us understand the core and evolution of Bambusa Arundinacea.

- *Despair supported wants to be*
- *Want of self-confidence support desires*

The above two rubrics form the core of Bambusa. We will understand these rubrics in depth and the connection of other rubrics with these ones.

Desire for support and want of self-confidence is the crux of Bambusa Arundinacea. The need for support is shown in different way. Sometimes the need for support is manifested as the patient goes from doctor to doctor to get treated. Another way the support is shown up needing to rest their body against the wall or chair, etc. The need of support can be the required during the financial crisis, emotional support from family, and much more. If Bambusa patients does not get support from his family, friends colleagues, etc they will develop physical symptoms like stiffness, and tightness in the extremities.

The main question comes here is why would Bambusa patients require support? Because such individuals has no ambition, they just grow aimlessly as Bamboo tree grows. They can perform routine task very perfectly but would not be able to show good performance for the new task. They develop anxieties due to lack of confidence prior taking any new tasks. To avoid any new task they would keep postponing the task. Additionally most of the time you will find them pessimistic about everything, hence they lose hope very easily, find themselves very helpless and goes into the state of indifference. Hence they want support all the time but cannot express the needs to their family.

How would Bambusa patients react if they don't get the required support? They will develop the physical complaints like stiffness in the back, headaches, heaviness and tightness in the body, etc. Other than physical symptoms, Bambusa patients will also develop anxieties and fear- *Fear of Failure, Fear of narrow spaces, Anxiety conscience, anxiety future about, anxiety health about and anxiety about money matters*. They also develop aversion towards everything in his life. They feels as if everything is restricted around him which makes him fearful for narrow place. Feeling of being caught in a life situation without having possibility to cope with it due to lack of support or tension.

Inability to handle family relations, inability to handle profession when it becomes demanding, inability to meet the financial needs of his family, etc. are the problems that arise if they don't get desire support.

Fear of failure is another critical aspect in Bambusa people. Why is the fear of failure so common in Bambusa patients? Bambusa personality has no ambition still they have strong fear of failure. This fear is due to lack of confidence. They people can perform the regular work vey meticulously, however they lack same meticulousness while performing the new task because they lack self-confidence.

These people are delusional as well. They have delusion as if their arms are stiff and life is cut off, delusion as if back is loosen and back is packed in streaks of fog. Feeling of forsaken is common as well. Feels as if he is alone in this world, no one to support him, hence his life is meaningless. He feels he is a failure, he fails in everything and he will not succeed in his life as he does everything wrong.

During physical complaints he feels as if his health is ruined, and he is going to develop some big disease like cancer. His health use to be fine but now nothing is right (delusion poor he is).

Conclusion

Need for support and confidence is the core of Bambusa Arundinacea. The anxieties, fear and delusional symptoms are all related to this core.

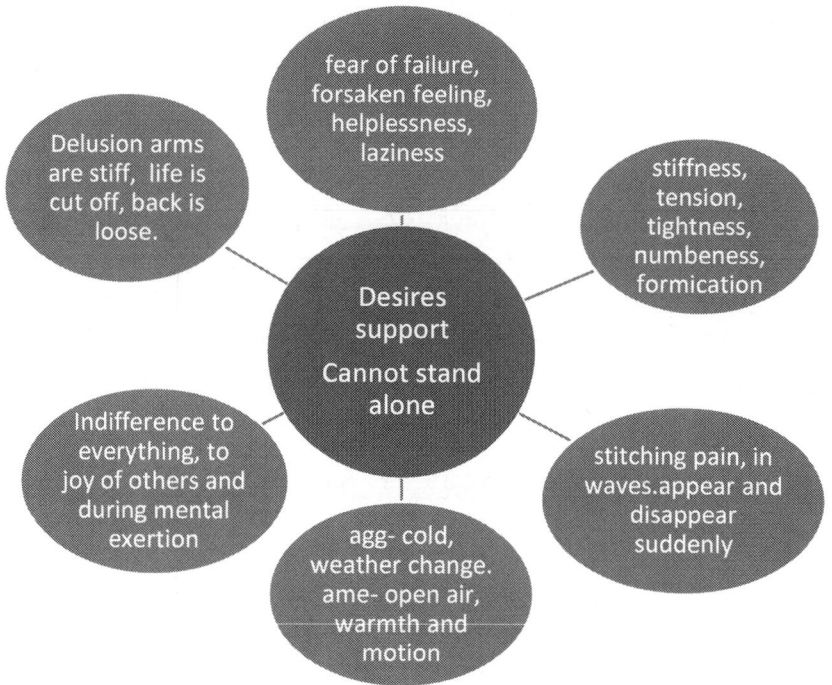

Crux of Bambusa Arundinacea

Reference:

Synthesis Repertory 9.1

Chapter 2: Sphere of Action

Bambusa Arundinacea acts on both mental and physical level. At physical level it acts on the bones, spine, and muscles. It has significant therapeutic action on Ankylosing Spondylitis also called as 'Bamboo Spine'.

Bambusa acts on endocrine system as well. Studies have shown that Bamboo has caused stimulation of endocrine systems especially gonadal functions, and to some extent on Thyroid functions. It is well indicated remedy for Pre Menstrual Syndrome and early menopause.

This remedy acts on neurosensory system too, however it has been rarely used for neurosensory problems. Neurosensory problems include paresis, paralysis, epilepsy, etc.

It acts on our metabolism too. It helps to stimulate the appetite, and digestion. Indicated in diarrhea and chronic dysentery.

Physical symptoms
Neck

There is a great tension and stiffness of the neck. The stiffness is so intense that it becomes very difficult to even turn the neck. This condition becomes worse from damp, cold weather and from being outdoors. The stiffness and tension can radiate into the arms as well. Along with the stiffness, there is intense pain that radiate down to the arm and extremities. Cramping and dragging kind of pain are usually present with stiffness. **The pains are better by rest and heat** which is an important modality of this remedy.

Extremities

Severe feeling of weakness and heaviness in the extremities which makes difficulty in writing and walking. Severe cramping pain with tension and stiffness in the lumbar and sacral region. Strong amelioration from warmth, heat and rest. Strong aggravation in the morning on waking, from cold and damp.

Another important symptoms are icy coldness of hand and feet with clumsiness and awkwardness. Sometimes along with the coldness of extremities, there can be burning of feet or soles.

Indicated in sciatica nerve pain, severe pain as if electric current running down the sciatica nerve to the hollow of the knee. Pain is so intense that the whole body shivers and trembles due to pain. Weakness from hip down to the knee as if beaten. These pains are worse by motion and better by pressure.

Back:

Bambusa is most commonly indicated in back and spine symptoms. Spine is primarily is affected in this remedy and has the referred effect on the extremities. Numbness and tingling begins in the back with radiation down to the extremities. Cramping, wave like pain is the characteristics of Bambusa remedy.

Head

Bambusa is commonly indicated in headaches where pain in the head is a referred pain either from back, spine or neck problem. Pressing pain in the head, feels as if band around the head. Heaviness in the head, desires to lean on something. Headaches are worse from physical exertion, cold wind, bending forward while feels better by rest in lying position.

Eyes

Although Bambusa is less frequently indicated for the eyes symptoms, one symptoms makes this remedy very peculiar. **Feels as if eyes are being pressed and pulled into the head, pressed from outside or pulled from inside.**

Nose

Dryness and numbness of nose with blockage in alternate nose. Sometimes watery discharge from the nose with sneezing. These symptoms sounds more of 'flu-like' symptoms. Very sensitive to the smell. Cannot bear any kind of smell, feels nauseous with the smell.

Throat

Great degree of roughness and soreness in the throat. Feels as if something is in the throat and has to clear the throat very often. Difficulty in swallowing anything. Sensation of a lump in the throat caused by accumulation of mucus in the throat. The mucus is difficult to hawk up. These symptoms again very similar to flu-like symptoms. Throat complains are markedly **relieved from hot drinks.**

Stomach

 Insatiable hunger or hunger with no appetite. Nauseous feeling. Strong aversion to fat and beer and also an aggravation from beer and wine. A desire for wine and cheese, for spicy food and for stimulants in general.

Abdomen

Severe bad smelling flatulence with severe pressure in the lower abdomen around and below the navel. Feels as if big bubble in the navel is moving. Diarrhea along with flatulence. Severe urge to pass the stool, cannot resist and has to go immediately. Stools are greasy and fatty. Diarrhea in the morning and mid night after 4 am. Diarrhea appears suddenly and disappears suddenly.

Chest

Sensation as if lump in the heart region. Stitching, burning pain and stiffness in the heart region. Worse by inspiration. Palpitation in heart with nausea, worse by lying on left side.

Sleep and dreams

Sleeplessness due to constant thoughts and activity of mind. Tosses and turns in the bed. Wakes up in the midnight between 3.30 to 4 am.

Female

Premature Menopausal remedy. Ailments from parturition. Leucorrhea white, offensive and watery aggravation before and after menses. Painful swelling of mammae. Headache before and during menses.

Mind symptoms

Bambusa has the strong mental picture. The mental symptoms of Bambusa revolves around the theme of Bambusa – Need for Support. The patient desires support from others that can be his family, friends, relatives, colleagues, etc. They desire change and freedom in their life, but unable to get it, hence becomes helpless, irritable, restless and depressed.

Bambusa patients are fearful too. They have fears like as if her conditions are observed by others (similar to Calcarea Carbonica), fear of poverty (similar to Arsenic Album, sepia), fear of failure, fear of impending disease, and fear of misfortune. Fear of failure is due to lack of confidence in himself. He can perform regular routine task perfectly however he would not be able to perform the new task, because he does not have confidence in himself. Hence he develops fear for failure. Due to this reason his family and friends will look down upon him. Family and friends blame him for his failure which ultimately hurts his honor. He cannot respond back to the people who blames him because of lack of confidence and lack of support. Hence Bambusa is associated with the ailments from wounded honor, suppressed anger, anticipation and fore brooding.

Anxieties are well marked in Bambusa remedy. Due to lack of support, they develop anxiety about future and money matters. After prolonged anxieties and sufferings they end up with feeling of despair. Despair of death with fear.

Bambusa patients develop several delusions during the illness. Delusion forsaken and alone in the world is also an important aspect of Bambusa remedy. The patient goes into the state of forsaken when he finds no support from others. He becomes loner. He feels helpless due to his ailments and hence feels as if he is poor.

Bambusa patients finally goes into the indifference but not as much as Sepia goes. During mental stress Bambusa patient becomes indifferent to everything. However he will apologize easily but Sepia will not. That's the difference between the indifference of Sepia and Bambusa.

Conclusion

In this chapter we learned the materia medica of Bambusa Arundinacea.

References:

Disease of Spine. Retrieved from:
http://www.anthromed.org/UploadedDocuments/diseases.o
f.the.spine.pdf.

Nick Churchill. A Reading of Bamboo. Retrieved from:
http://www.homoeopathie-
online.com/materia_medica_homoeopathica/bambus.htm.

Chapter 3: Bambusa Arundinacea Homeopathic Proving

This chapter will describe the homeopathic proving of Bambusa Arundinacea. Thanks to Bernd Schuster who brought the new remedy into light by proving it on different provers.

This chapter will list down the proving symptoms of Bambusa Arundinacea. The symptoms are mentioned in the patient's original words. These symptoms are taken from Bernd Schuster proving.

The goal of this chapter is to precisely understand the symptoms described by the provers which ultimately will help us to understand the theme and crux of this remedy.

Bambusa was proven in 1994 by Schuster in Germany. There were 20 provers, and as a result, 2000 new symptoms were added to The Complete Repertory.

Emotional and Mental Proving Symptoms

- Want to sleep naked
- Inclination to take the medicine again
- Feeling that time passes too quickly
- Thinking less about sex
- Cry out because of the intense pain in the middle of the sole of my right foot.

- Depression with a "fear of poverty" when walking outdoors
- Depressive thoughts.
- Keep thinking about our financial future.
- It weighs on my mind that cash is always so tight.
- I worry, I'd really like to run away.
- Bouts of depression with idleness again at 4.00 p.m.
- I wonder what's going to happen.
- Shattered and tired at 2.00 p.m. Can't straighten things out.
- I've no idea what to do with myself
- At 4.00 p.m. anxious about not being able to deal with what's in store for me over the next few years.
- There's just a huge mountain of things to overcome.
- Everything seems uncertain to me.
- Feeling I can't manage makes me incapable of doing anything at all.
- Fairly sad for 2-3 hours (1.30 p.m.) without being aware of any precise reason. Don't want to have anything to do with anybody. Morose.
- Sad at 4.00 p.m.
- Depressed, feel I'll never be well again.
- Want to make everything perfect, don't want to hurt anybody.
- Feelings getting all mixed up again.
- Feel deserted and betrayed.
- Depressed when there is no work
- It hasn't bothered me over the last few weeks.
- Emotionally very sensitive, I feel inferior in some way, can't help crying over trivial things. Feeling sorry for myself. No-one asks if they can help me. Feeling lonely. Better again by the evening.

- Very sad, weeping a lot at night. I feel deserted. I never feel I can wholly depend on my wife. I find too much closeness in the relationship suffocating. Knowing this causes me deep pain.
- Still very sad, but more hopeful than yesterday.
- Feel as if my "emotional foundations" are lacking. I say something and feel that what I am saying is not quite right because I am not in touch with my feelings at that moment but more on the surface.
- It is like a separation between emotion and intellect.
- Again the sense of not having any emotional attachment to certain things. It is as if there is something missing. Have no involvement with a lecture I am preparing.
- Feel hurt by some harmless comment yesterday evening.
- Think I am starting my mid-life crisis.
- Very touchy and vulnerable all day.
- Feeling of pointlessness.
- Listless, cannot get round to doing anything (in the morning).
- Feel irritable, weak and feeble. Better for rest and fresh air.
- Tendency to moan.
- Better during the day, worse at night.
- Depressed when there is no work.

Physical Symptoms of Proving

- Very difficult to turn the neck
- The stiffness is really very intense, 'like a poker'
- A wave of pressure coming from my abdomen upwards to my throat
- Feeling of burning along the spine as if heat comes in waves
- Right hand is thicker than her left
- A totally unfamiliar heaviness of the limbs on waking
- An extreme feeling of coldness starting from the shoulders and radiating downwards
- Feeling of heat in the feet although I was objectively cold.
- Dropping things and bumping into things when walking
- Feeling of a foreign body in the shoe
- Painful electric currents running down the sciatic nerve to the hollow of the knee. So intense that the whole body trembles and shivers
- Could hardly walk in the morning
- Weakness from the hip down to the knee as if beaten
- Feeling of a band around the forehead, as if pressing from inside outwards.
- Pain like a stick in the back of my head
- I feel like death, I just want to rest, I don't want to see or hear anything
- Feeling of the nose as if tickled by a feather
- I am sensitive to smell like a pregnant woman
- Skin felt very thin, something an old person might feel

- Feeling as though a big bubble in the navel was moving around
- The pressure around the waistband
- Flatulence come out like a fire hydrant, like a gush of water
- Constantly turning ideas over in the mind
- Want to sleep naked and run around naked
- Want cool fresh air
- Depressed with no real interest in life.
- Don't want to go out, want to be left alone.
- Helpless feeling, tearful, depressed, black despair.

Conclusion

Some mind and physical proving symptoms taken from Bernd Schuster proving are mentioned in this chapter.

The proving symptoms indicates the exact physical and mental symptoms of the provers.

Reference

Bernd Schuster. *Bamboo Homeopathic Proving of Bamboo Arundinacea Repertory and cases*

Chapter 4: Bambusa and Other Differential Remedies

In this chapter we will learn how to differentiate Bambusa with other similar remedies. This differentiation will help you to understand the remedy more clearly and able to differentiate it in your practice. The physical and mental symptoms of Bambusa resembles closely to other remedies.

Remedies that closely resemble Bambusa are: Silicea, Rhus Tox, Sepia, Staphysagria and Cimicifuga

Silicea

Like Bambusa, Silicea is a mild and yielding person. Silicea is an obstinate personality, when they are under stress they perform their best and shine as they are intelligent people. However they lack stamina. They cannot sit for longer time, and get tired easily.

Silicea is mainly indicated for skin, bones and muscular complaints. Similar to Bambusa, Silicea is a chilly remedy, hence symptoms are developed from cold and damp weather.

Like Bambusa, if Silicea had to perform any unusual mental task, they develop fear of failure due to anxiety to perform well. However ultimately they perform well. Silicea does not need support like Bambusa needs, however

Silicea lack confidence which leads to physical and mental complaints.

Rhus Tox

Rhus Tox mainly acts on the fibrous tissues, joints, and tendons. Strain on the muscle, over lifting and cold damp weather are the reason for developing the symptoms. There is severe pain, stiffness and swelling in the joints. Most of the pains are better by motion and lying on hard surface and aggravated by rest, unlike Bambusa where pains are better by rest and heat. However cold damp weather aggravation is present in both the remedies.

Restlessness is marked feature of Rhus Tox. Restlessness is associated with all its complaints. Hence joint pains are relieved by movements or motion. They cannot sit at one place for more than few minutes before getting up for a short walk or stretch. They are unable to sleep at night as they constantly toss and turn whole night. Waking up in the morning is very difficult due to morning stiffness and inflexibility of joints. Once a little flexibility is restored to the joints, the pain lessens considerably and they can continue their restless search for comfort through the day.

Similar to Bambusa, Rhus Tox has severe stiffness associated with the illness. *Rhus tox is helpful when initial movement is painful and stiff, however the continue motion eases the pain.* This is very important feature of Rhus Tox which will help the practitioners to differentiate Bambusa from Rhus Tox. In Bambusa, the pain and stiffness will remain the same even with the continued motion. There will be no relief from continued motion.

Emotionally Rhus Tox is unbendable, it has the tendency to hold back, finds difficult to respond others. At the end, when they are worn out by the pains, they turn into fixed ideas and superstition.

Sepia

Sepia is very similar to Bambusa at emotional level. Indifference towards everything, aversion towards children, irritability towards children, desire to escape, helplessness feeling, and discontented feeling are present in both Bambusa and Sepia. However the core of Sepia is different than Bambusa. Sepia suffers when her freedom is restricted. Sepia performs her duty very well with respect to housekeeping, raising children, as a caring and nurturing woman and a mother, however she needs to liberate herself from this traditional mould. Hence she develops helplessness feeling and indifference towards everything especially towards her husband and children. Sepia goes into indifference after long run of battle however Bambusa loses hope immediately due to lack of support from others. Bambusa is less indifferent remedy than Sepia.

Like Sepia, Bambusa is also considered as 'Women Remedy'. Sepia mainly acts on the venous circulation of female pelvic organs. Hence 'stasis' (caused by venous circulation) is commonly seen at mental and physical levels. On physical level, stasis of uterus leads to prolapse of uterus. Muscles become weak due to loss of control by the autonomic nervous systems. Similarly at emotional level, stasis or stillness of emotions is seen. She has feeling without emotions ultimately leads to indifference. She remains in this state of indifference for a very long time, while Bambusa does not go and /or remain into deep state of stasis and indifference.

Sepia is markedly ameliorated by violent motions which distinguishes Sepia from Bambusa.

Staphysagria

Bambusa and Staphysagria shows similarity on an emotional plane. Both develop the symptoms after suppressing their anger, hence both remedies are present in the rubric, Ailments from, anger suppressed. However understanding the reason for suppressed anger will help us to differentiate both the remedies. Staphysagria suppressed the anger because he/she does not want to wound their honor by expressing their anger, they want to be a 'nicer person' in front of people's eye so they get fame from others. Bambusa has suppressed anger because of lack of self-confidence and does get enough support from his environment (family and relatives).

Staphysagria has ailments from wounded honor, mortification and indignation. Staphysagria has great indignation about the things done by others or herself. These patients get easily angry but rarely manifest the anger because they are afraid of losing their image in front of others. They lack ability to express their feelings. Hence they develop physical ailments like headaches, menstrual irregularities and glandular affections.

Bambusa's honor gets wounded when no one supports him and when his family starts neglecting him. Bambusa also suppresses the anger which is manifested in the form of stiffness and pain in the extremities.

Kalium Phosphoricum (Kali Phos)

Kali Phos very closely resembles Bambusa as one of the core of this remedy is desire for support. Kali Phos patient are usually very weak, easily tired and prostrated kind of. Most of the complaints arise due to over exertion, over work, grief and worries. *Slightest exertions seems to be a heavy task and fades away all energy.*

Similar to Bambusa, Kali Phos goes into the state of indifference, where he becomes indifferent to her family and surroundings. Along with indifference these patients goes into the state of insanity and weakness of mind. Here comes the difference between Bambusa and Kali Phos. Bambusa would not go into the state of insanity.

Kali Phos is a great nerve remedy hence act well in nervous complaints. Complaints related to weak memory, forgetfulness, hurriedness in action and speech, and over sensitiveness especially to noise are predominant features of this remedy.

Cimicifuga Racemosa

Cimicifuga is mainly indicated in muscular complaints, complaints related to uterus and ovaries and rheumatic complaints.

Sensation of cloud enveloping her is the main indication of Cimicifuga. They feel as if dark black clouds has enveloped her, and hence something bad is about to happen to her.

Cimicifuga is well indicated in stiffness in neck and back muscles. The stiffness and pains are very similar to the

Bambusa, however in Cimicifuga, pains are rheumatic in nature.

During each menstrual flow, they suffer from 'labor like pain', pain becomes more with increase in flow. Great debility between menses. Hysteric or epileptic spasms at the time of menses. In Bambusa, neuralgia is less as compared to Cimicifuga.

Cimicifuga is also a great remedy for headache but the headache is of uterine origin (in Bambusa headache is due to spinal stiffness) due to great rush of blood to head; the brain feels too large for the cranium. This congestion to head is the effect of suppression of uterine discharges or suddenly ceasing of neuralgic pains. It is felt in the eye balls and is increased by the slightest movement of the head and eye balls. This headache is better in open air.

Reference:

James T Kent. Homeopathic Lecture on Materia Medica.

Chapter 5: Bambusa Case Studies

In this chapter we will gain deeper understanding of Bambusa through practical cases. This chapter includes three cases of Bambusa with follow ups.

Case 1: Ankylosing Spondylitis

Ms A.K, 30 year old married woman came with the severe pain and stiffness in the lower back. She had been suffering from Ankylosing Spondylitis for 5 years and since then has been taking prescribed medications, however there was no improvement or complete cure of AS with these medications. The pain and stiffness would return back as soon as she stops taking the medicine. Her treatment included pain killers (Tab. Paracetmol 500mg thrice a day for first few years, later he was prescribed for Ibuprofen 200 mg twice a day) and steroidal doses during unbearable attack of pain.

Here is the conversation with this patient:

Dr: What's your problem? How can I help you?

Patient: I have severe pain in my lower back. I cannot move, walk, sit or even stand due to this pain. Also I feel stiffness in my back, feels as if there is some kind of tension in the back. It remains stiff all the time, especially in the morning after waking up. This has been going on for last 5 years.

The pain travels from lower back to both the hips till the legs. Also feel numbness and tingling in the legs.

Dr: What things aggravate the pain and what does ameliorate it?

Patient: Any kind of motions like walking, sitting, or even standing makes this pain severe. I feel better only by lying down and by taking rest. Also hot water bath relieves me for time being. I sit in hot water bath tub every day after taking shower.

Dr: What else happens due to this pain? How do you manage your routine life with this kind of pain?

Patient: My sleep is unrefreshed all the time because I wake up in the middle of night or early morning around 3 am and cannot fall asleep. I have become irritable due to this pain.

Dr: Tell me more about your nature and about yourself.

Patient: I got married 4 years back. I have a 2 years old daughter. My husband was very supportive to me during the initial 2 years after marriage. He used to help me manage household work during the time of severe lumbar pain. But now he has been neglecting me. We live with my mother in law and father in law. My in-laws taunt me for not being able to perform the household work. I want to do everything correctly but this stiffness stops me from doing anything. No one is able to understand me. Whenever they taunt me, my husband just listens and says nothing. I don't get support from him at all. I would feel better if at least he would say something against them and support me. But that never happens. This upsets me a lot. Hence I get very angry at my husband and daughter, but later feels guilty.

I also want to pursue my career. I have done Bachelors in Communication, I am interested in pursuing further education. But my husband doesn't support me, he says first manage the home and then think about studies. He has been neglecting my interests and my passion. I need emotional and financial support from him but he doesn't understand that.

Recently I noticed that I have been losing confidence in everything. I use to speak very confidently with strangers but now I have lost that confidence, feels that people might be noticing me, feel I will fail in everything, I will fail in my studies, my career and even in personal life. I have lost hope from my life. I dwell constantly on these thoughts. Hence I avoid taking any new task, I either neglect new tasks or postpone working on that.

Case Analysis:

Along with physical complaints, her emotional state was more concerning to me. Throughout the case she was complaining that her husband not being supportive. Lack of support from her husband is her main concern. Also she lacks confidence to do anything in her life. She has been neglecting and postponing her work as well. Hence she was looking for support in the form of career and education.

Need for support and lack of confidence is the main theme of this case, which is also the core of Bambusa remedy.

Based on above analysis, following rubrics were taken from Synthesis 9.1 repertory:

Mind, fear failure

Mind, confidence want of, support desires

Mind, postponing everything to next day

Mind, helplessness feeling

Bambusa 30c, two doses were prescribed for two days.

Follow ups

After first prescription, she called me to tell that after 5 years she has been relieved from back pain. Mentally was feeling calm too. However her confidence level and concern for support from her husband was still present.

Bambusa 200c single dose was prescribed which showed drastic improvement in the back pain. Numbness and tingling in extremities were significantly reduced.

Over the period of time Bambusa 0/2 made her emotionally confident. She no longer complained about her husband's and in-laws behavior. She pursued her further education with great confidence.

Case 2: General Weakness

A 50 year old man complained of general body weakness since 3 months. He work as a security guard in an apartment complex. He has 2 sons, eldest son is jobless while younger son is disabled. He said, 'he is unable to do his work properly. I always feel tired, weak and lazy'. No history of any major chronic illnesses like Diabetes Mellitus, Hypertension or cardiac problems.

Dr: How do you manage your routine work?

Patient: It is very difficult to manage my routine. I don't feel like doing anything. Hence I feel irritated on my wife and children.

Dr: Is there any tension or thoughts that's troubling you?

Patient: I have two sons but both are not helpful and supportive to me financially. Eldest one is jobless, he use to does some fir but recently left the job. He never took care of household expenses when he was earning. Younger son is disabled since last year as he had major accident. I am struggling financially. I have to manage the medical bills for my younger son and also household expenses.

I have postponed purchasing my medicines. Due to these thoughts I feel depressed all the time. I never feel like going to work. I am tired of struggling alone, I have 2 sons but never got support from them. Feel like going away from all these worries.

Case Analysis

This case clearly shows that there is the strong anxiety about finances and about future. Also shows the need for support as he expects his sons to support him. Lack of this support has made him physically and mentally weak.

Based on the analysis, following rubrics were considered for further evaluation of the case.

- Despair, supported wants to be
- Anxiety future about
- Anxiety money matters about

Bambusa 200c single dose was given.

Follow ups

After a week he smilingly said that he is much better, he feels energetic as he used to be before. Also he started morning walk for about 30 minutes without any weakness.

After a month same remedy in same potency was prescribed when he had similar episode of weakness. The same potency took care of his complaints very well He is still taking care of his disabled son but this time without any complaint. Since last follow up he has been doing well.

Case 3: Postnatal Depression

This is a case of 32 year old female who developed stiffness in the back with pain in left leg and depression after pregnancy. Along with this major issue she had been also suffering from frequent headaches.

Her description about her problems clearly indicates Bambusa. However during first consultation, I incorrectly considered her as 'Sepia'. She was better with Sepia however her complained were not completed gone. After closer understanding about her problem, Bambusa strike to me and worked miraculously on her overall health. Here is the description of her complains in her own language.

Dr: How can I help you?

Patient: 3 months back I delivered a baby girl. I had no problem throughout the pregnancy and during delivery as well. However after delivery, I started getting severe headaches, and lower backache. Backache is so severe feels as if stiff and tense. The pain from lower back goes to left leg. It's pretty much like a sciatica pain. This pain is relieved by lying down or sitting in a chair. I cannot stand or walk for a long distance. Since last two months I have been suffering from headaches which comes at least once in a week, feels better after taking painkiller relief is only for a time being.

The most important thing I am worried is my nervous breakdown. I don't feel lively and energetic. I am very caring for my baby but not able to take proper care of her. Recently I have become very irritable, and express my frustration on my baby. Sometime I weep without any reason, I never cried before but now I cry most of the time. I get very anxious for my baby and her future.

Dr: How did it started? Can you relate any event that triggered or started this behavior in you?

Patient: Around 8 months of pregnancy, my husband lost his job, depression started since then. I started getting anxious about my baby, how will I take care of my baby, how will I feed her and what can I do solve this problem? He is jobless till now. He does some menial work to get the money, but there is no guarantee of his earning. I feel so HELPLESS. Wish I could work somewhere. I want to earn money for my family but I cannot move, I feel I am so stiff, cannot move anywhere. So helpless.

This all happened because of my husband. He never took his work seriously. He never took any responsibility of the family. I had to always work hard and make earnings. I thought he had changed hence I left my job, but situation is still the same. This makes me very angry.

The lower back pain and headaches started soon after delivery. I assume these complaints are related to my worries and depression. If something happens to me no one would take care of my baby. I have no parents, and no close family, some few friends but not sure if they can be any help to me. I am so alone in this world. She started weeping while describing this point.

Case Analysis
The mental symptoms are more critical than physical symptoms. All her symptoms started when her husband lost his job, as she lost support from her husband which she had been always expecting from him. Additionally she decided to resign from her job so she could concentrate on her pregnancy and baby. Since she has no support from her

husband and other family members she has gone into nervous breakdown and has the strong feeling of being helpless and alone in this world and assumes that there is no one who can support her. She is in the state of despair.

These thoughts and anxiety are so strong that she developed severe stiffness in the back, sciatica pain and recurrent headaches.

Based on the analysis, following rubrics were considered of further evaluation of the case.

- Delusion, blames her partners bad mood, she is
- Despair, desires support
- Helplessness feeling
- Delusion alone being in the world
- Despair supported wants to be
- Weeping, forsaken feeling from

Bambusa 30c single dose for 2 days was prescribed.

Follow ups

Within a week stiffness in the back reduced drastically, however headache still persisted.

Further few repetitions of Bambusa 200c the headache was completely gone within a month. Back pain and sciatica almost gone. The most amazing result was shown at mental level. She accepted her husband as he is. She had no resentment for her husband, she thinks now that her husband supports her.

Her husband started working at a startup company and has a decent salary. Also anxiety regarding the future of her baby and herself is no more. She has been living happily as a small family.

Case 4: Pre Menstrual Problems

This is a case of 25 years old lady who complained of severe headache and tenderness in the mammae before menses. She has been suffering from this problem since menarche. However the problems has been increasing since 3-4 years.

Dr: Can you describe your complaints in detail?

Patient: I get severe headache before menses and lasts till the 3rd of menses. The pain is so severe that my head gets tightened which constricts the neck muscles. During this episode I get severe stiffness in the neck as well. Neck stiffness is related with the headaches.

Other than headache, I have been also suffering from heaviness in the breast area, especially before and during the menses.

Dr: What are the things that aggravate the headaches and breast tenderness? What you do to ameliorate these symptoms?

Patient: Usually they get aggravated before menses. Headaches get worse when I am tense and thing too much about somethings. I really don't feel fine until I pop up painkillers.

Dr: Do you get any other problem during, before or after menses?

Patient: I do get pain in lower abdomen during menses. Pain is severe for first 2 days, then gradually lowers. Feels better only by sitting against the wall. I cannot walk or lie down during the pain.

Dr: Tell me something about yourself.

Patient: I got married 4 years back and we live in a joint family. I have a very hectic life. I have to manage my work life and personal life. I work part time in a company. Since I live in a joint family and I am the youngest daughter in law I need to take care of every one. Before marriage my life was hectic too. I use to work three jobs – 15 hours every day. Financially I was not doing well so had to work extra hours. Even after marriage I have been going through same physical work which makes me tired all the time but I never give up. I wake up every day and continue my routine. Husband is never there for me. Even after doing so much for this joint family no one even ask me if I need any help from someone. This is too much now. Even with all these problems I manage to do my office work meticulously. I never give up on the work, will work hard to get it done.

Case Analysis

This young lady is mainly tired of being overworked, she needs some change and help from people around her. She expects her husband and in laws to help her out but they don't provide her support and help she needs. This is her main concern which needs attention. Also her physical complaints get worse before menses is striking too.

Based on analysis, following rubrics were taken into consideration.

Rubrics taken from Synthesis Repertory:

- Mind responsibility, responsibility taking too seriously
- Mind Desires Support
- Head, pain accompanied by, Neck pain in
- Head pain, menses before agg
- Chest, Tension mammae, menses before

Bambusa 200c single dose for three days was prescribed (remedy was taken a week before the menses)

Follow Ups

A week after the first prescription, she mentioned that during this cycle she noticed less intense headaches. She was able to do her work even with headaches. Heaviness in the breast was still the same during the cycle. Mentally felt bit calm.

Bambusa 1M single dose was prescribed a week before the menses. This time her cycle was free of pains, very mild headache and tenderness in breast. Also there was no pain in abdomen during the menses which was not the case before. She also said my in-laws are getting along with me. They try to help me out whenever I ask them. Now mentally I am stress-free.

She needed 1M single dose once in 5 months or so. She has been doing well till now.

Case 5: Cervical Spondylosis

47 yrs women came with the complaints of neck pain radiating to both the arms was accompanied by her daughter. X-ray reveals mild cervical spondylosis. Throughout the conversation patient looked sad and depressed.

Dr: What's your problem? How can I help you?

Patient: I have severe pain in neck (showing her neck) I have taken physiotherapy and allopathy medicine but no relief. Pain radiates to both the forearms till the fingers. Sometimes I feel my fingers are numb. This problem started 4-5 years back, but since couple of months it has increased.

Dr: How do you manage the pain?

Patient: I take pain killer and just lie down when there is pain leaving the work aside. I don't have any other health issue, eveyhting is normal except this neck problem.

Dr: Who all there in your house?

Pt: My son, daughter and my husband.

Dr: Any problem in your house?

Patient: she waited for seconds and said yes Dr, my husband had major business loss thereafter he is not working at all and started drinking too. Till our business were good there was no problem for me.

My son goes to college but he does not study properly. My daughter goes to school.

Dr: How are you managing financially?

I have started small catering business where I prepare and deliver food. During marriages or other events I get lot of food orders but nobody is there to help me out. I prefer to deliver the food on time but both my husband and son are not helpful. My daughter is young she tries to help me out. Sometimes my friends come for help. Most of the time I am alone managing this business.

Her daughter said she is the only one who takes care of our house. She is the one who pays our school and college fees.

Dr: Your husband won't help u?

Patient: no Dr, he will roam around and asks money for drinking and gambling. I have no other option than giving him money or else he will get so angry and will shout

Daughter said that my mother cries at night after we all slept, many times I have waked up and consoled her.

Dr: any other complaints?

Patient: Showed her palms, had cracked skin with mild bleeding from cracks. No other health problem. I want this neck pain to be cured as soon as possible so that I can do my routine work and earn money so that I run my family peacefully.

Case Analysis

This lady seemed to be very depressed and sad throughout the conversation. She is the only earning member of the family, should pay fees for both children. Husband is not at all support financially.

She weeps all the time and daughter has to console her.

Rubrics from Synthesis Repertory

Mind, Anxiety about money matters.

Mind, Weeping - forsaken feeling, from – night

Mind, Confidence - want of self Confidence - support desires.

Mind, Fastidious - perfect way wants to perform in a

Bambusa 30C three doses a day for 2 days was prescribed.

Follow Ups

Neck pain was reduced by 60% in 3 days. Mentally she was feeling calm and better. She was relieved from pain for 15 days. However the complaints relapsed after that, Bambusa 30 c repeated with gradual increase to 1M potency. She remained stable for significant amount of time on higher potency. Never had to change the remedy even for acute complaints. All her complaints were settled with the single remedy.

Conclusion

In all the above cases, every patient had issues with finances and lack of desired support. Their ailments started when they did not get the support from their loved ones. After taking Bambusa, not only the physical complaints drastically reduced but also they improved mentally and emotionally. Mentally they became strong and positive, able to handle the situation and face the hurdles without any concern. This is the beauty of Homeopathy. It not only treats your ailments but make you a better person who is able to adapt the life situations.

References

Synthesis Repertory 9.1

Made in the USA
Las Vegas, NV
11 January 2022